In praise of Edward de Bono

'Edward doesn't just think. He is a one-man global industry, whose work is gospel in government, universities, schools, corporates and even prisons all over the world' *Times 2*

'The master of creative thinking' *Independent on Sunday*

'Edward de Bono is a cult figure in developing tricks to sharpen the mind' *The Times*

'Edward de Bono is a toolmaker, his tools have been fashioned for thinking, to make more of the mind' *Peter Gabriel*

'de Bono's work may be the best thing going in the world today' *George Gallup, originator of the Gallup Poll*

'The guru of clear thinking' *Marketing Week*

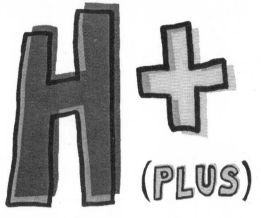

A NEW RELIGION?

H+ (PLUS)

How to live your life positively through
Happiness, Humour, Help, Hope and Health

Edward de Bono

Vermilion
LONDON

1 3 5 7 9 10 8 6 4 2

First published in the United Kingdom in 2006 by Vermilion,
an imprint of Ebury Publishing
Random House UK Limited
Random House
20 Vauxhall Bridge Road
London SW1V 2SA

Random House Australia (Pty) Limited
20 Alfred Street, Milsons Point, Sydney,
New South Wales 2061, Australia

Random House New Zealand Limited
18 Poland Road, Glenfield,
Auckland 10, New Zealand

Random House (Pty) Limited
Isle of Houghton Corner Boundary Road & Carse O'Gowrie, Houghton, 2198,
South Africa

Random House UK Limited Reg. No. 954009
www.randomhouse.co.uk
Papers used by Vermilion are natural, recyclable products made from wood grown in sustainable forests.

A CIP catalogue record is available for this book from the British Library.

ISBN: 0091910471
ISBN 13: 9780091910471 (from January 2007)

Printed and bound in Australia by
Griffin Press

Copies are available at special rates for bulk orders. Contact the sales development team on 020 7840 8487 or visit www.booksforpromotions.co.uk for more information.

H+

Human+

Happiness+

Humour+

Help+

Hope+

Health+

Is H+ a religion?

... Maybe.

Is H+ different from other religions?

... Maybe.

Is 'maybe' a good
enough basis?

… Maybe.

Most religions focus
on the ultimate 'truth'.
There seem to be
different versions of this.

Maybe 'maybe' is also useful.

BELIEF

Many religions have a belief in the supernatural. This may be a belief in God or in supernatural forces. Some ask for a belief in many gods.

In H+ there is only a belief in the potential of yourself and in the potential of your fellow human beings. H+ sets a framework for the development of this potential. You believe that you can act in a certain way or that you will eventually be able to act in this way.

COMPATIBLE

H+ is a way of life that is fully compatible with any other religion or framework: Christianity, Islam, Judaism, Hinduism, etc.

H+ does not impinge upon or compete with other belief systems.

You can keep all the beliefs and values of those other religions and simply add H+ to them.

H+ provides an 'action framework'. Although action frameworks are implicit in many religions, they are not as explicit as in H+, which is based on action.

This action framework can be added to any existing religion or belief system since there is no contradiction at all.

DIFFERENT

Most religions focus on avoiding sins and wrongdoing. With H+ the emphasis is entirely on positive action. You have to contribute and make a difference. Being free of sin is not enough. The emphasis is on action and involvement with the world. Many religions suggest detachment from the world and the peace of tranquillity. With H+ there is action and achievement. Your self-worth arises from your achievements, not from meditation.

There is no intrinsic belief system in H+ except the belief in yourself – not necessarily as you are but as you can be. At the same time any belief system belonging to any other religion is fully acceptable. This is unlike most religions, that do not tolerate other belief systems.

A WAY OF LIFE

H+ is a religion in the sense that Buddhism is a religion.

H+ is a way of life.

Maybe we should invent a new term of 'woligion' to cover 'a way of life religion'.

POSITIVE AND NEGATIVE

Most religions emphasise the negative.

Most religions tell us what we should not do. There are defined sins and guilt and punishment – even in eternal fire.

H+ is entirely positive. The emphasis is not on sins that are to be avoided but on things that are to be done.

The original purpose of the negativity of most religions was to keep order in society by ensuring that people behaved in a suitable way. H+ uses the negativity that is already in place from laws, other religions, moral precepts, social behaviour, etc. All these continue to operate in the same way. To them is added the positive nature of H+.

In H+ the emphasis is on:

POSITIVE

CONSTRUCTIVE

CONTRIBUTING

In H+ it is not enough to detach yourself from the ills of the world. It is not enough to sit in a corner and perfect yourself. You perfect yourself only by contributing to your fellow human beings and the world around.

You help yourself by helping others. There are no hermits in the desert unless they are thinking big thoughts that will eventually help others.

The intention of helping others and the effort of helping others is what matters. The effectiveness of that help may need to be developed over time.

Every 'plusser' (which may become the general term for those who know about H+) will have a private agenda of actions that could help others.

You assess yourself on how successful you have been in helping others.

There is emphasis. There is attitude. There are actions. The emphasis on certain matters leads to the development of specific attitudes. These matters are listed in the following pages and are all part of the H+ framework.

Then there are the actions. There are no sins as in most religions. Instead there are positive actions. When these are carried out they develop a sense of achievement, an increase in self-esteem and the habit of contributing – instead of being self-centred and passive. These positive actions are called 'pons'. Their role and nature will be described later (see page 54).

HUMAN+

H+ stands for Human+. The 'plus' indicates the best or positive aspects of humanity. There are also well-known negative aspects, such as fear, violence, aggression, deceit, etc.

There is, for example, hatred. In the H+ framework, the only thing you hate is hatred itself.

Just as there is no doubt that humans can be very nasty creatures, so there is no doubt that humans can also be wonderful creatures. The emphasis is on the positive aspects.

There is no wish that people should be perfected robots. On the contrary, they should be even more human – but on the positive side.

There will be lapses, failures and deflations of positive energy. But there is hope that the negative phase will come to an end and the plus factors re-establish themselves.

HAPPINESS+

Happiness is also central to H+. Happiness needs to become a deliberate habit and not just the feeling when everything is perfect.

For too long literature has encouraged the idea that tragedy, disaster, despair and anguish are the true stuff of life. Everything else is seen as trivial and superficial.

Every town has a hospital and every hospital has an emergency department into which accident victims are brought. There is plenty of agony, tragedy and despair. Do we go and sit in those emergency departments for entertainment or to learn about life?

It is true that unhappiness is an important part of life, but so is happiness. The media tend to celebrate disaster, criticism, wrongdoing and scandal because that is the easy way to arouse interest. It requires rather more skill to arouse interest from happiness. It is also that the media, rightly, sees its role as the conscience of society, that should expose defects and failures.

Maybe there should be a 'happiness rating' for movies. There could be an HH film or even an HHHH film. Viewers would know in advance that they were to going to see a 'bang-bang' shoot-out or a neurotic ballet of emotions.

There is more truth in happiness than in despair.

Happiness is not just the absence of pain and suffering. Just as we need to value things and to become more sensitive to value, so we also need to foster happiness in a deliberate manner, for example by seeking out those things which make us happy.

Thinking is very important for happiness, because with thinking we take charge of our lives instead of being like a cork in a stream pushed around by the currents. Thinking can change our perceptions and these control our emotions. Thinking can provide us with ways of doing things and solving problems. Thinking can enable us to understand other people and to get on with them. Thinking has been shown to reduce crime dramatically in young people.

CoRT stands for Cognitive Research Trust. This is a programme of thinking lessons that is now widely used in schools all around the world. The lessons are aimed at broadening and enriching perception. Very simple tools can be learned, used and become a habit. For example, the OPV (Other People's View) encourages the thinker deliberately to explore the thinking of another person. Once this is done, many conflicts just disappear. The C&S (Consequence & Sequel) encourages the thinker to look at the immediate, short-term, medium-term and long-term consequences of a choice or action. Doing this deliberately is very different from believing that you do it. One group of very senior executives was asked to assess a suggestion. Eighty-six per cent were in favour of the suggestion. They were then asked to do a formal C&S. The percentage in favour dropped to just 15. Yet every one of the executives would claim that his or her job demanded a constant look at consequences.

Happiness is very much to do with expectations. There are expectations that the world and other people should treat you in a certain way – and unhappiness when this is not the case. There are expectations that you should achieve something and unhappiness when your talent or circumstances fall short of your aim.

Happiness should be the natural state and unhappiness an interruption, just as a cold or a headache are interruptions in your normal state of health.

Adjust and change

If you learn to adjust to the present situation, you may be happier about it. Failure to adjust has no advantage.

It may be claimed that if you adjust too well you will not try to change the situation. But it is only an assumption that adjust and change are opposites. You can adjust and continue to seek change at the same time. The motivation for change does not have to be your unhappiness, but the will to change and make things better.

A 'proto-truth' is a truth that we hold to be true so long as we are seeking to change it.

Happiness is a matter of attention. If we get into the habit of focusing attention on negative aspects, we are likely to be unhappy. If we learn to focus on more positive aspects, we can be happier. A young woman was born without legs but seems to be a happy person. She takes part in athletics and is a catwalk model.

Usually our attention is pulled or drawn by things around us. If we develop the habit of 'directing' our attention where we want to, the habit of happiness becomes easier.

Thinking and happiness

Society has paid far too little attention to thinking. This is unfortunate because thinking is the most fundamental human skill and determines both our happiness and our achievements.

Our traditional thinking habits are based on recognising a standard situation and providing a standard answer. They are 'judgement' based. Then there is argument, logical deduction and 'proving that you are right'. All this is excellent, just as the front left wheel of a motor car is excellent – but it is not enough.

We have neglected to develop constructive thinking; creative thinking; perceptual thinking; and design thinking. You can analyse the past but you have to design the way forward.

Judgement brings the past into the future. Design brings the future into the present.

Critical thinking is never enough when you need design to put together what you have to deliver, the values you want.

Over the years I have developed various frames and methods of thinking that are now widely used in thousands of schools and hundreds of organisations around the world.

Instead of argument, there is the method of 'parallel thinking' to explore the subject (with the 'Six Thinking Hats'). One corporation that used to take 30 days on their multinational project development now does it in two days. A small Canadian corporation reckoned they saved $20 million the first year they used the method.

There are also the 'Six Action Shoes', dealing with styles of action. The 'Six Value Medals' provide a frame for value scanning.

Then there are the formal creative methods of lateral thinking based on an understanding of the brain as a 'self-organising information system'. These tools can be powerful. Using just one of these tools, a group of workshops in South Africa generated 21,000 ideas in a single afternoon.

Then there are the ways of improving perception incorporated in the CoRT programme, that is widely used in schools throughout the world. Teaching this programme for just five hours to unemployed youngsters in the UK (the Holst Group) brought a 500 per cent improvement in the employment rate. In Australia, Jennifer O'Sullivan taught these methods to unemployed young people who were completely deaf – and achieved a huge increase in employment.

Young people who have been told by schools that they are stupid find that they are not stupid at all but can think and take control of their lives. Their self-esteem rises and everything else follows.

There is a close relationship between thinking and taking control of your life and happiness. This is not 'thinking' in terms of philosophical intellectualising, but simple, practical thinking tools and methods that can be used equally by Nobel prize laureates and young people with Down's syndrome. Teaching thinking to unemployed young people increased the employment rate five fold. Teaching thinking to young people too violent to be taught in mainstream schools reduced the rate of criminal convictions to one tenth (compared to those not taught thinking).

Some religions appear to discourage people from thinking and prefer them to act out of faith and belief. This may make sense, since much thinking may be confusing and misleading. With H+ you are encouraged to think – even if you are wrong.

Habit

Happiness is an intended habit – just like dieting. You may fail from time to time, or even most of the time, but you just keep on trying.

HUMOUR+

No religion emphasises the importance of humour. Buddhism in general and Zen Buddhism in particular emphasise the need to change perceptions. This is indeed how humour works but the emphasis in Buddhism is not on humour, as such, and its role in human behaviour and human society.

It may be that humour was seen as a danger to the solemnity of most religions.

Yet humour is a key lubricant of life. Humour is a social glue. Humour is the best anti-arrogance device. Humour is the best anti-despair device. Humour is what may separate man from other creatures. So why is humour neglected?

Whether you offer other people something to laugh at, or whether you laugh at what others offer, it is a form of generosity. You are interacting in a way that is not threatening, not demanding and not serious.

Lightness of being and lightness of touch are key aspects of H+.

Humour develops the habit of mind of seeing things in different ways, of exploring possibilities. Humour dilutes the certainty that is the basis of so much emotional anguish. You can learn to laugh at yourself as well as at others.

Anything that can be threatened by humour deserves to be threatened.

Humour is not funny.

Humour is very serious.

Humour is about not taking the world or ourselves too seriously.

Our brains like certainty. Perception seeks certainty. We then lock on to that certainty with rigidity, arrogance and intensity.

Humour is all about the possibility of looking at things in a different way. Humour is all about the possibility of changing perceptions.

In humour we change perceptions and suddenly see that the new perception makes logical sense.

Humour is about lightness. This is the opposite of intensity, seriousness and anguish, that lock us into negativity.

Humour is a social lubricant because it is a way of inter-acting generously with people. In humour we share the possibility of a new perception with others. With humour we give to others and yet lose nothing ourselves.

What was the evolutionary benefit of humour? Why does a supposedly superior species have a sense of humour? How did that help with survival?

Research by David Perkins at Harvard showed that 90 per cent of the errors in ordinary thinking (not high tech) were errors of perception. Perception was limited, egocentric, short term, etc.

The ability to change perceptions and to look at things differently probably had a high survival value. Humour itself was a by-product of that ability.

Attitude

Humour is an attitude, not just the ability to tell jokes.

If someone sets out to insult you and you shrug and do not feel insulted, then you are not insulted.

Humour is a way of cutting the puppet strings that sometimes make us hostage to the world around us.

Humour replaces certainty with 'maybe' and possibility. Maybe we could look at this differently.

When there are things that need to be taken seriously, we choose to take them seriously – but can retain the lightness of humour.

Humour builds self-esteem. You are not at the mercy of the world around you because you can laugh at it.

Instead of asking someone to 'lighten up', we can get into the habit of asking a person to 'press your humour button'.

Humour is central to H+ because that is the only way we can take it seriously.

HELP+

This is the fundamental principle of H+.

Why?

Research in the USA showed that 94 per cent of young people rated 'achievement' as the most important thing in their lives.

How do you get achievement?

You may be a great sports star. You may be excellent at exams. You may set up a successful business. You may become a rock star.

All these are possible and provide a great sense of achievement.

But what about day-to-day achievement?

What about those who are not going to be sports stars or successful entrepreneurs?

Most religions have sins of one sort or another. Sins are all about the bad things you should not do. But is it enough not to do bad things? With H+ there are 'positive sins'. These are things you should do. They are positive actions ('pons', see page 54) of help to others and to the world – daily acts of help or contribution that provide the opportunity for multiple small achievements. You set yourself an agenda of pons, no matter how small they may be, and you get a sense of achievement through doing them. From achievement comes self-esteem and a belief in yourself.

You help yourself very directly by helping others.

The importance of these small acts of help, or pons, is that they have a clear objective. If you help an old lady across the road, it is clear that you have done this. Achievement is visible. If you preach to a group of people, you can only hope that you have helped them.

HOPE+

There are few things sadder than the suicide of a young person. In Australia the most common cause of death in people under the age of 24 is suicide. This may be because Australia keeps better suicide statistics than other countries, where suicides may be hidden for religious reasons.

The suicide of an elderly person is no less tragic but is more understandable. A person may have tired of the world or run out of the will to live. The person may be in pain from a terminal illness. But for young people there are no such reasons.

A quarrel with a boyfriend or girlfriend, failure at an exam, low self-esteem can all lead young people to believe that the future has nothing to offer.

Hope is key. During the Second World War, prisoners in concentration camps faced appalling conditions. Many of them kept up their hope over years until they were finally liberated.

There is hope that appalling conditions will pass, no matter how black and permanent they may seem at the moment.

There is hope that you will adjust yourself to the conditions and no longer be bullied by them.

There is hope that, through your own efforts, things will get better.

Even when hope is completely deluded, it is always worth having hope. That is not to say that you neglect to indulge in daily work because one day you may win the lottery.

With the hope in H+ you seek to make things better. You also learn to 'shrug' and become less of a hostage to the world around.

In many religions, prayer is a form of hope. You pray to God to make things better and believe that in his wisdom God may do so.

There is passive hope and there is active hope where you seek to take action to make things better.

You can also contribute to making things better for others.

I wrote a book – *Tactics: the art and science of success* – based on interviews with successful people in various walks of life, from entrepreneurs to sports people. There were huge differences in style and personality between the people interviewed. Some were impulsive, others were careful planners. Some were bold, others were timid. The one thing that was common to all was the expectation of ultimate success. Problems on the way were just obstacles to be overcome. That is a very powerful form of hope.

HEALTH+

Health is also a key component of H+. With health you may be concerned, sensible, obsessional or even fanatical. That is entirely up to you.

The main point is that you pay heed to health as an aspect of your being a human being (Human+).

Health is a baseline on which everything else is built. If you are not healthy you are not able to help others and may absorb help that could be better used elsewhere.

If you owned a motor car you would bother to put fuel in the tank. You would bother to put air in the tyres. If you are capable of being healthy, it seems careless not to try to be healthy.

So a concern for health is as basic to H+ as a concern for happiness.

COOL

In a primary school in England, the day before Guy Fawkes Day, a six-year-old had drawn a picture of Guy Fawkes about to blow up the Houses of Parliament. Guy Fawkes was labelled as being 'cool'.

Guy Fawkes was about to blow up the Houses of Parliament and kill many people. This behaviour was not very moral. But the apparent style of what he was doing led to the young girl calling him cool. This separation between the nature of the action and the style in which it is done is the basis of cool. There is an obvious danger in the approval of the style and the ignoring of the nature of the action.

In schools all over the world, children want to be cool. It is claimed that cool came from American slave culture. The only form of power available to slaves was personality power. This meant being disdainful, your own person, confident and unflustered by the world around you. Through jazz and other means, cool entered our culture.

Cool has no moral aspect at all. As long as you do something with style, that is cool. Films and television programmes depict cool gangsters.

In school, cool means stylish: wearing the right clothes and belonging to the right clique. It means being confident and being your own person. In general it means 'good'. Surprisingly, there is no other term for 'good'. No one wants to be a 'goody-goody' so cool has a clear field.

Warm form

The coolest person around is a corpse. The corpse is independent and untroubled by the world around. The corpse is actually very cool. The corpse contributes nothing.

As a style, cool is defensive and contributes nothing. It is very ego-centric. It is a detachment from the world.

'Warm form' is the opposite. Warm form means that you are so confident that you can afford to be outgoing and generous. You smile whether people smile back or not.

Waffo

This is the usable term for warm form. If you are 'waffo', it means that you are generous, warm and human. You contribute to others and the world around. Unlike the cool corpse, you are up and about.

Will waffo replace cool? Probably not. But it can provide an alternative idiom – which at the moment is lacking.

Waffo and H+

There is no direct connection between waffo and H+. Waffo exists in its own right, separately from H+. Waffo is used here as an illustration of the attitude underlying H+. It is an outgoing, contributing attitude rather than a cold, self-centred one. With H+, you help yourself by helping others.

It is not a 'bargain'. You help others because you want to. You do not help others only if they help you. The sun shines even if no one worships the sun any more.

It is important that the background attitude of H+ be fully understood. H+ is not a 'belief and worship' structure. You do not behave in a certain way because you fear punishment if you do not behave in that way. H+ is directly a behaviour structure. You come to want to behave in a certain way. This is first. You then change as a result of the behaviour.

H+ is all about doing.

There is a famous quote from the French philosopher René Descartes:

Cogito ergo sum.
(I think therefore I am.)

There is another quote from Edward de Bono:

Ago ergo erigo.

(I act therefore I construct.)

H+ is about action.

'PONS'

H+ is based on action and contribution. A 'pon' is a positive action. You may help an old lady across the road. You may teach a child to read. You may clear up rubbish in your neighbourhood. You may intervene to help a mugging victim.

H+ is more than thinking good thoughts and having good intentions. H+ requires positive action that makes a positive difference in the world around you – or the world at large. For this reason, pons are central to H+.

A pon is a real action designed to help other people. This would usually be in the immediate local surroundings, but a wider area is not excluded.

A pon is simply a 'positive sin'. Just as a sin is something you are not supposed to do, and about which you are encouraged to feel guilty, so a pon is something you are supposed to do and about which you are encouraged to feel proud.

You can boast of your pons to yourself and to others. They are achievements.

Most religions encourage meritorious acts. Here contributing actions are the very basis of the religion. That is how you build up belief in yourself.

Agenda

A pon is a positive sin. That means an action that is helpful, constructive and contributing.

If you pick up a piece of waste paper and put it into a dustbin, that is a pon.

If you help someone who is confused and lost at an airport, that is a pon.

The agenda is the number of pons you set yourself as a target for the day. This could also be described as your quota.

Pontoon

A pontoon is a series of boats placed across a river so that you can get across the river. Here a 'pontoon' is the series of pons you place to carry you through the day.

You need to keep the same number of pons for every day.

You may choose to change the number occasionally, but in general you stay with the chosen number.

You should never have fewer than two pons in your agenda. You may have as many as you like, but realistically four would be a reasonable limit.

Pons are usually not planned in advance. You may, however, choose to place yourself where there are more opportunities for pons. There are times when it would be appropriate to plan a pon in advance.

Beggars

If you give money to a beggar, is that a pon? If you have an agenda of four pons and you give money to four beggars, are you achieving your quota of pons?

The answer is no for two reasons. The first reason is that it is too easy. There is no sense of achievement. You are just fulfilling an obligation in the easiest possible way. This will have little effect on yourself.

The second reason is that it may be antisocial behaviour to encourage begging by providing beggars with an unearned source of income.

Charities and good works

There are people who are already involved in charities and good works. How does this fit in with pons and constructive behaviour?

Ongoing good work is worthwhile and to be recommended, but it is not the same as individual, spontaneous pons.

The point about pons is that they are separate acts of help and contribution. This means that there will always be an attitude of readiness to help and to contribute. The habit develops, encourages and reinforces such an attitude. If you are engaged in a worthwhile programme, that is of immense value, but it is not the same thing.

So being involved in charities and good works and giving money to beggars are not pons.

Pons are small, spontaneous acts of help and contribution.

H+ recruitment

If you let others know about H+ by talking to them or by sending them a copy of *H+ (Plus) A New Religion?*, is that a pon?

Yes, this would indeed be a pon. But this sort of pon should never make up more than half of the pons on your agenda. So if you have an agenda of four pons a day and you recruit three people, that only accounts for two pons out of your agenda of four.

The reason is that behaviour, no matter how worthwhile, should not remove the need for spontaneous acts of help – and the readiness and attitude that goes with these.

What is important about pons is the immediate sense of accomplishment and achievement. It is not enough to be on the right road. You must be able to pick individual daisies from the roadside as you travel.

It is not just a matter of *being* a good person. You must be a person doing good things.

It is very important that this fundamental aspect of H+ be fully understood.

It is not the usual approach, that says that a good person does good things.

It is almost the opposite: you discipline yourself to do good things and so make yourself a good person.

Being asked for help

Once it becomes known that you are willing to help, people may start coming to you for help. This would be the case in a small community and less so in a larger one.

How should you react?

Does responding to a request for help constitute a pon?

How you react is very much a matter for individual judgement. How you respond to requests for help depends on your assessment of your time and commitments and whether the requests are genuine or just using your generosity.

What is important is that responding to such requests does not constitute a pon. This may seem unfair and contradictory, because responding to requests may actually be more helpful than thinking up your own pons.

Just as giving money to a beggar is too easy a form of contribution, so may be responding to requests. There is none of that proactive readiness to contribute that is the basis of H+. Reactive responding is highly valuable but is not the same as proactive initiatives and actions. There may be no difference to the person receiving the help, but there is a big difference to the person offering the help. It is the difference between being passive and being active.

THINKING UP PONS

This is more difficult than it may seem.

Once you have the right attitude, you will come to see more easily and more often opportunities for pons.

In time, individuals may build up a repertoire of types of pons and will see those opportunities in places where others may not see them.

Boasting sessions may also suggest new pons that others have used.

Over time, a catalogue of pon suggestions will develop on the Internet. You can then access this catalogue if you are completely out of ideas.

The most important part is to develop a readiness to help, a readiness to see opportunities for pons. This readiness is as important as the actual carrying out of the pon. It is more important than the mechanical carrying out of a pon that has been suggested on the Internet.

You can set your mind to designing pons for future use. They can be as imaginative as you like. Always keep in mind that pons are small and separate acts of help. They are not a single major task. That may be worth doing, but the separateness of the pons, each from the other, is important to give repeated small achievements and to keep open the readiness of mind to contribute and help. Major projects are very worthwhile but are not substitutes for individual pons.

BOASTING AND SHOWING-OFF

There is nothing in H+ to stop you being proud of your achievements.

You should keep a specific H+ diary and list your daily achievements.

Through the Internet you can connect up with a 'boasting buddy' and exchange details of your achievements.

With or without the Internet you can join up with a group of others. You might meet occasionally, in real life or on the Internet, to exchange and compare your achievements.

If this boasting comes to provide a motivation for your behaviour, there is nothing wrong with that at all. If the ultimate behaviour is helpful and contributing, the initial motivation is unimportant. In the end, all help is motivated by personal reasons.

The important thing about pons and agendas is to show yourself that you are capable of the discipline of H+, capable of finding pons and capable of achievement.

There is nothing better for self-esteem than achievement.

Pons provide a daily source of small achievements. That benefits you directly.

At the same time, each pon benefits others directly or indirectly.

FAILURE, FINES AND ACHIEVEMENT

You set your own agenda or 'pontoon'. If you find that you cannot cope with a larger number of pons on your agenda, you can reduce the number to just two. That is a matter for your confidence in yourself.

What happens if you fail to carry out the pons on your agenda? Does that matter?

It does matter. It matters so much that your failure must somehow be turned also into an achievement.

If you fail to carry out your self-assigned pons, there is a penalty. The penalty is a fine.

Just as you choose the number of pons on your agenda, you also choose the fine for each unfulfilled pon.

You could set a fine of 1p for each unfulfilled pon. If you have an agenda of four pons a day and never carried out any of them, that would cost you £14.60 over a year.

In this way assessing and paying the fine also becomes a form of achievement.

You choose the fine. If you are more confident, you could set a pound for each unfulfilled pon, or even £10. That is entirely up to you.

You may wish to accumulate the fines before sending them. The fines should be sent to H+ central headquarters (see page 85 for address).

The intention is that the fines will be used to finance the organisation of H+ and for educational purposes. This is not, however, a guarantee. The fines may be used for purely frivolous or personal purposes. This is important, because if you felt that paying the fine was simply contributing to a worthy cause, then the fine means very little.

There has to be some disappointment and pain in paying the fine.

Paying the fine is the ultimate opportunity for achievement and discipline. If you have not been able to carry out your self-directed pons, how do you get a sense of achievement? You get this sense of achievement by formally paying your fine. If the fines were only to go to charitable purposes, then the motivation to carry out the pons would be much weakened in favour of making a charitable donation (which is very much easier). The fine is much more powerful if you resent paying it because there is no guarantee that it will be used only for charitable purposes. This aspect is a key part of the value of the fine.

Ideally, you should never have to pay any fine. You set your own agenda or pontoon and then carry out the pons. That is your sense of achievement. That is the basis of your belief in yourself as having the discipline to do what you want to do. At any time that you feel the H+ framework and discipline are not providing you with something useful, you can simply drop out.

PROJECTS

The individual acts of help and kindness called pons are central to H+. You are what you are because of the way you act. Being saint-like and selfish or detached is not what H+ is about.

Projects are not central to H+ but are entirely optional. Through local contacts, or through the Internet, you might set up a project team. You decide on a task and then use your thinking to plan how to carry out that task. In general, tasks should be helpful to others and contribute to the world around you.

One possible framework for such tasks is the 'YEAH team'. This is a project framework that was set up for young people:

Young

Energy

Action

Help

A booklet available from the Edward de Bono Foundation in Dublin (see page 93) lays out the steps and the framework.

Any other framework would do as well.

Pons are lonely acts, and there are times when people want to bond and to work with others. Projects are a way of doing this.

Projects, actions and successes can be written up on the Internet and so shared with others.

Projects provide an opportunity for thinking, planning, motivation, action, social interaction – and a sense of achievement.

To repeat: projects are not essential to H+ in the way that pons are essential. Projects are never a substitute for individual pons. A project, no matter how worthwhile or involving, never removes the need for daily pons.

RITUALS

Many religions are festooned with rituals. At first sight these seem silly and superfluous. Taken each on its own, rituals may seem pointless.

Yet rituals seem to be very important. Some of the older religions have strong rituals that may contribute to their strength.

The value of a ritual is that it involves self-discipline and belonging. The ritual is pointless in itself so the doing of it is purely a matter of discipline and the willingness to do it. It is an active affirmation of your belonging. The ritual is a visible signal to yourself and to others that you belong, in some way, to a group. Each time you carry out the ritual you are saying to yourself, 'I belong'.

A ritual is a mechanical way of affirming that you belong. Even if your spirit is not inspired or even enthusiastic, the ritual carries you along. Furthermore, ignoring or rejecting a ritual is a definite act of defiance that most people are not prepared to make.

There is another value to rituals. This is the discipline of carrying them out even when you do not want to and even when you think they are pointless.

It is for these reasons that H+ has one ritual.

In the morning, before doing anything else, you take a sheet of paper. On this sheet you draw 100 circles. These circles may be of any size or regularity. They may be the same or different in size. The circles may be arranged in neat rows or scattered randomly. That is your choice. You may vary your arrangement from day to day. Put a date on the sheet.

This is a boring, pointless ritual. That is exactly the value of the ritual. The discipline of doing it when you see no point in doing it gives it its value. That is the same value that translates into carrying out pons.

You can carry out this ritual every day. To make it more difficult, you are only required to do it for four days a week. You now have to choose when you do it and to remember when you have done it.

This ritual is specifically designed to be pointless, but disciplined.

SIGNALS

There may be times when you want to signal to someone else that you follow the H+ concept.

You may want to identify other people like you in order to exchange experiences or simply to talk to someone with whom you have something in common.

There is a discreet hand signal which could be helpful.

With your right index finger you touch the right side of your nose. If the other person responds by doing the same, then you take the same right index finger and touch the outer corner of your right eye.

If you are on the receiving end and you see someone touching the side of his or her nose, you need to check whether this is intentional or just chance. So you touch the side of your nose as well. Then, after a pause, you touch the outer corner of your right eye. If the other person follows, there is a good chance he or she knows about H+.

You may choose to use such signals as you wish or not at all.

ORGANISATION

Energisers

Energisers are individuals who put energy into the H+ framework and who provide care and organisation for those who use the framework. Anyone can choose to be an energiser.

An energiser recruits people to take up H+. An energiser, if he or she wishes, sets up a team of H+ users. The energiser acts as a communication source.

Because H+ can be added to any existing religious acceptance, people already involved in different religions can add H+ to their activities and become active H+ energisers in addition to whatever else they are doing. H+

provides a framework for behaviour that is positive and contributing. This should have a value in many areas.

The energiser collects the fines of the people in his or her team. Sixty per cent of the fine is retained by the energiser and 40 per cent is sent to central headquarters (see page 85).

An energiser may set up sub-energisers to amplify his or her efforts. In such cases the energiser allocates part of the energiser's share of the fine to such sub-energisers as he or she wishes.

The energiser can organise meetings or groups or projects but is not permitted to add anything to the basic H+ message without specific permission from headquarters.

Fines

If a low fine is being paid it makes sense to allow this to accumulate into a larger sum. Fines are paid either to central headquarters or to the local energiser who has recruited you. No one is obliged to deal with the local energiser unless he or she wants to. If the local energiser has recruited you, it makes sense to work through him or her. There is, however, no 'area franchise'. Different energisers may be working in the same area.

Where an energiser passes on the allocated part of the fine to headquarters, the name of the person paying that fine must be given – not just a sum of money.

COMMUNICATION

This will be mainly, but not exclusively, via the Internet:

www.hplusanewreligion.org

www.edwarddebono.com/hplus

In addition, there may, from time to time, be mail or other means of communication.

Although the Internet is frequently mentioned in this book, it is by no means necessary. You can operate within the H+ framework and make no use of the Internet at all. You may have no knowledge of the Internet or no ability to use it, but you can still make full use of the H+ system. You may obtain information directly from the net or through your local energiser, if you have one.

REGISTRATION

Every member of H+ should be registered centrally unless there are particular reasons for not wishing to be registered (see opposite for contact address).

In time, members of H+ may be invited to join special circles or groups depending on their energy, effectiveness and interests. Such circles will be announced from time to time.

HEADQUARTERS

There are two headquarters:

Central headquarters

This is the heart of the H+ framework. Policy, procedures and changes all come from central headquarters. All fines are paid to central headquarters, either directly or through the local energiser.

Dr Edward de Bono
P.O. Box 5075
London
W1A 0WW
United Kingdom

Operational headquarters

This is the 'management' of the H+ system. This headquarters deals with administrative matters, enquiries, organisational details and so on.

From time to time operational headquarters may pass matters on to central headquarters, but enquiries should first be sent to operational headquarters via the Internet:

www.hplusanewreligion.org

www.edwarddebono.com/hplus

or the address shown on page 85.

Information, books and products can all be obtained from operational headquarters.

It should be understood that, depending on the volume of mail and enquiries, it may not be possible to respond to all communications in a direct way.

SUMMARY

H+ stands for:

Human+

Happiness+

Humour+

Help+

Hope+

Health+

This book – or framer – sets out the basic principles of the H+ religion (way of life). You may follow the system rigorously, partly, sporadically or weakly. The decisions are left to you at all points.

The elements of H+ are fully compatible with any belief system, religion or social structure.

The emphasis is on the positive rather than the negative.

The emphasis is on action and contribution rather than personal purification.

The emphasis is on small constructive and contributing actions rather than other forms of worship.

The emphasis is on building self-esteem through repeated achievement. The achievements are small but the cumulative effect can be large.

The emphasis is on helping others in order to help oneself.

At all times the emphasis is on the 'plus' or positive side of humanity. Goodness is not just the absence of badness but an active contribution.

H+ requires no more from you than a belief in the potential of yourself and the potential of your fellow human beings. This is a belief that you can contribute to the world around you in the way you act. The framework of H+ sets out a way in which you can get a sense of achievement through positive action. This is the basis for self-esteem.

ABOUT THE AUTHOR

Edward de Bono is the leading authority in the field of creative thinking and the direct teaching of thinking as a skill. While there are thousands of people writing software for computers, Edward de Bono is the pioneer in writing software for the human brain. From an understanding of how the human brain works as a self-organising information system, he derived the formal creative tools of lateral thinking. He is also the originator of 'parallel thinking' and the Six Thinking Hats. His tools for perceptual thinking (CoRT and DATT) are widely used in both schools and business.

Edward de Bono's instruction in thinking has been sought by many of the leading corporations in the world, such as IBM, Microsoft, Prudential, BT (UK), NTT (Japan), Nokia

(Finland) and Siemens (Germany). The Australian national cricket team also sought his help and became the most successful cricket team in history.

A group of academics in South Africa included Dr de Bono as one of the 250 people who had most influenced humanity in the whole course of history. A leading Austrian business journal chose him as one of the 20 visionaries alive today. The leading consultancy company, Accenture, chose him as one of the 50 most influential business thinkers today.

Edward de Bono's methods are simple but powerful. The use of just one method produced 21,000 ideas for a steel company in one afternoon. He has taught thinking to Nobel prize winners and to young people with Down's syndrome.

Edward de Bono holds an MD (Malta), MA (Oxford), DPhil (Oxford), PhD (Cambridge), DDes (RMIT) and LLD (Dundee). He has had faculty appointments at the universities of Oxford, Cambridge, London and Harvard and was a Rhodes Scholar at Oxford. He has written 70 books with translations into 40 languages and has been invited to lecture in 58 countries.

The Edward de Bono Foundation is concerned with the teaching of constructive thinking in Education and Management. For further information contact:

The Edward de Bono Foundation
PO Box 2397
Dublin 8
Ireland
Tel: +353 1 8250466
Email: debono@iol.ie
Website: www.edwarddebonofoundation.com

ALSO AVAILABLE FROM VERMILION BY EDWARD DE BONO

How to Have a Beautiful Mind	9780091894603	£8.99
The Six Value Medals	9780091894597	£8.99

FREE POSTAGE AND PACKING

Overseas customers allow £2.00 per paperback

TO ORDER:

By phone:	01624 677237
By post:	**Random House Books**
	c/o Bookpost
	PO Box 29
	Douglas
	Isle of Man IM99 1BQ

By fax: 01624 670923

By email: bookshop@enterprise.net

Cheques (payable to Bookpost) and credit cards accepted.

Prices and availability subject to change without notice.

Allow 28 days for delivery.

When placing your order, please mention if you do not wish to
receive any additional information.

www.randomhouse.co.uk